Mediterranean Diet Cookbook for Kids

Discover Vibrant and Flavorful Recipes for Healthy Eating

Carrie Richard

Table of Contents

INTRODUCTION

Dear young chefs and culinary adventurers, This cookbook was created just for you; it is full of tasty recipes, vibrant ingredients, and fascinating culinary adventures that will not only pique your interest but also support the development of your developing body and mind.

The Mediterranean Diet is a way of life that is praised for its many health advantages and the delight of enjoying real, fresh food. It is not only about diet. This diet is a celebration of nature's abundance and gastronomic variety, including the cuisines of nations around the Mediterranean Sea, such as Greece, Italy, Spain, and others. It is not a rigorous regimen.

We encourage you to delve into a range of recipes in this cookbook that highlight the key components of the Mediterranean Diet: colorful fruits and vegetables, whole grains, legumes, lean meats, healthy fats, and fragrant herbs. We hope that these recipes will open your eyes to a world of tastes and encourage well-balanced eating practices that improve your health in general.

Why the Mediterranean Diet?

Not only is the Mediterranean Diet well-known for its delicious food, but it is also praised for its many health advantages. This diet, which is high in minerals, antioxidants, and healthy fats, has been associated with a lower risk of heart disease, obesity, and several types of cancer. Furthermore, it's important to promote family dinners and attentive eating practices in addition to what you consume.

Eating like people who live near the Mediterranean is about living a certain way as well as the cuisine. It promotes having unhurried mealtimes, enjoying meals with loved ones, and appreciating the preparation and enjoyment of food. It is our aim that this cookbook will serve as an inspiration for you to make delectable meals and then enjoy them with loved ones, making treasured memories around the dinner table.

What This Cookbook Is Expecting

You'll discover a variety of recipes in these pages that have been thoughtfully chosen to appeal to adventurous souls and youthful palates. There's something for every mealtime and appetite, from hearty breakfasts to filling lunches, tasty dinners, and delicious sweet indulgences. Every dish is created with the convenience of use in mind, so you can help out in the kitchen of course, under the supervision of an adult.

To aid you through every step, we've also included a ton of photographs and useful advice, so cooking will be not just tasty but enjoyable and instructive as well. You will find nutritional statistics next to the recipes to help you comprehend the amount of goodness that goes into each meal.

Are you prepared to go on this gastronomic journey now? Take off your apron, put on some sleeves, and join me as we explore the colorful world of the Mediterranean Diet, where every dish combines health and enjoyment.

Benefits of the Mediterranean Diet for Kids

As parents, caregivers, and educators, we all want what's best for our children. Enter the Mediterranean Diet a treasure trove of health benefits specifically tailored for kids. It's not just a diet; it's a lifestyle that champions wellness, and its benefits for young ones are nothing short of remarkable.

First and foremost, the Mediterranean Diet is a powerhouse of nutrients essential for a child's growth and development. Packed with fresh fruits, vibrant vegetables, whole grains, and lean proteins, this diet provides a smorgasbord of vitamins, minerals, and antioxidants. These super nutrients are superheroes for growing bodies, boosting immunity, and aiding in healthy development.

One of the standout features of this diet is its emphasis on heart health. The inclusion of heart-healthy fats like olive oil, nuts, and fish works wonders for young hearts, promoting cardiovascular health from an early age. Omega-3 fatty acids found abundantly in fish are like superheroes for brain development, supporting cognitive functions and helping kids excel in school.

Let's talk about the fuel for energy carbohydrates! The Mediterranean Diet offers a balanced intake of whole grains, providing a sustained source of energy. This means kids can power through their busy days without the dreaded energy crashes.

Weight management? Check! Studies show that following the Mediterranean Diet reduces the risk of childhood obesity. The abundance of fiber-rich foods helps kids feel full and satisfied, curbing unhealthy cravings and promoting a healthy weight.

It's not just physical health; mental health also thrives on this diet. The consumption of nutrient-rich foods is linked to improved mood, focus, and overall mental well-being in children. The joy of cooking and sharing meals with loved ones fosters positive relationships and a healthy attitude towards food.

But wait, there's more! The Mediterranean Diet isn't just about what's on the plate; it's a lifestyle that encourages physical activity and family bonding. Kids who grow up embracing this lifestyle are more likely to maintain healthy habits as they grow older, setting the foundation for a lifetime of wellness.

The Mediterranean Diet isn't just a diet it's a recipe for a happy, healthy, and vibrant childhood. It's a feast of benefits that nourishes the body, fuels the mind, and sets the stage for a lifetime of wellness.

CHAPTER 1: THE MEDITERRANEAN DIET EXPLAINED

What is the Mediterranean Diet?

The Mediterranean Diet is a way of life-based on the eating customs and culinary traditions of nations surrounding the Mediterranean Sea, including Greece, Italy, Spain, and southern France. It goes beyond a conventional diet. Nutritionists and other health professionals have examined this eating pattern in great detail due to its many health advantages.

The mainstay of the Mediterranean diet is an abundance of foods that are derived from plants, such as whole grains, legumes, fruits, vegetables, nuts, and seeds. Olive oil serves as a main source of fat and is substituted for butter or other fats in cooking and dressings.

Essential elements of the Mediterranean diet are:

- **Fruits and vegetables:** They provide vital vitamins, minerals, and antioxidants and are the cornerstone of the diet.

- **Good Fats:** The main and most common source of monounsaturated fats that are good for you is olive oil. Nuts and seeds are sometimes included as well, adding even more beneficial fats.

- **Whole Grains**: Consuming whole grain products such as bread, pasta, rice, and other grains daily helps to provide fiber and nutrients.

- **Lean Proteins:** A moderate diet of chicken, eggs, dairy products (such as yogurt and cheese), and fish and shellfish are recommended. Red meat is only sometimes eaten.

- **Herbs and Spices:** A lot of herbs and spices are used to flavor food, which means less salt is needed.

- **Modest wine Consumption:** Although it's not required and should only be done by adults, several Mediterranean diets recommend a modest amount of red wine with meals.

The Mediterranean diet's focus on whole, minimally processed foods and the inclusion of a range of nutrient-dense selections is one of its important features. It also encourages a well-rounded way of living that incorporates social interaction, consistent exercise, and mindful eating.

The Mediterranean diet has been associated in several studies with several health advantages, such as lowered risks of heart disease, stroke, certain malignancies, and increased lifespan. It is an excellent option for anyone looking for a balanced and health-supporting diet because of its nutrient-rich content and emphasis on fiber, healthy fats, and antioxidants.

Nutritional Advantages for Kids

The Mediterranean Diet is a nutritional treasure trove designed specifically for children, providing a plethora of health advantages that support their general development, growth, and well-being.

Above all, this diet offers an abundant source of vital nutrients, including a diverse range of vitamins and minerals that are vital for children's development. The main components of this diet, fruits, and vegetables, are high in minerals like potassium and magnesium as well as vitamins A, C, and K. These nutrients are essential for maintaining strong bones, teeth, and an immune system that keeps children healthy and able to fend off infections.

Fish, almonds, and olive oil are good sources of healthy fats that are essential for children's growth. Fish is a great source of omega-3 fatty acids, which are particularly important for brain health and cognitive function. They improve learning, memory, and focus. Additionally, these fats aid in the nervous system's growth, which guarantees that children develop to the best of their intellectual and social abilities.

Children may benefit greatly from whole grains, which are another essential component of the Mediterranean diet. Because they include complex carbs, which assist in maintaining stable blood sugar levels and avoid energy crashes, they provide a prolonged source of energy. Furthermore, the fiber in whole grains helps maintain a healthy digestive system and keeps youngsters feeling content, which lowers the chance of them overindulging in harmful snacks.

Lean protein sources like fish, chicken, and lentils are included to make sure children get enough protein for growth and muscular development. In addition, the Mediterranean Diet lowers consumption of saturated fats by favoring plant-based proteins over red meat, which over time improves heart health.

Additionally, a strong immune system is supported by the quantity of antioxidants found in colorful fruits and vegetables, which protects children from common infections and diseases.

The Mediterranean diet for children is, in essence, a nutrient-rich treasure trove that promotes healthy growth, cognitive development, and immunological strength rather than merely being about mouthwatering tastes. Kids may start along the path to a healthier, more promising future by adopting this nutritious eating habit.

Importance of Balanced Eating

The cornerstone of a healthy lifestyle is balanced nutrition, which acts as a compass to direct people especially children toward the best possible growth, development, and general well-being. It's important to embrace a wide variety of nutrients that serve as the building blocks for a healthy body and mind rather than focusing just on what's on the plate.

Fundamentally, adopting a balanced diet entails ingesting a range of foods in appropriate amounts from various food categories. Fruits, vegetables, entire grains, lean meats, dairy products, and healthy fats are all included in this. Every one of these dietary categories contributes a different combination of macronutrients, vitamins, and minerals that are essential for different body processes.

In particular, a balanced diet is crucial for developing children. It gives them the nutrition they need to support their quick formation of bones, fast growth, and cognitive abilities. Foods high in nutrients support their energy levels and provide them the attention and endurance needed for academic pursuits as well as physical activity.

Furthermore, a balanced diet develops healthful eating habits at a young age, laying the groundwork for lifelong excellent health. Encouraging children to learn the benefits of a balanced diet helps them make better food choices as they become older by instilling in them the necessity of fueling their bodies with the correct foods.

Additionally essential to the prevention of illness is a healthy diet. For example, antioxidants from a diet high in fruits and vegetables help fight oxidative stress and lower the risk of chronic illnesses including diabetes, heart disease, and certain types of cancer.

Moreover, maintaining a healthy connection with food is promoted by balanced eating. It promotes mindful eating by emphasizing savoring meals and paying attention to your body's signals of hunger and fullness. This strategy aids in the prevention of bad eating practices including undereating or overeating.

Eating a balanced diet involves embracing a broad range of nutrient-dense foods that promote optimum health and feed the body, rather than adhering to rigid diets or restrictions.

CHAPTER 2: BREAKFAST DELIGHTS

Rainbow Fruit Yogurt Parfait

Ingredients:

- Greek yogurt (1 cup)
- Strawberries (sliced) (1/2 cup)
- Blueberries (1/2 cup)
- Raspberries (1/2 cup)
- Honey or maple syrup (2 tablespoons)
- Granola (1/4 cup)
- Optional: Chopped nuts (almonds, walnuts) (2 tablespoons)

Instructions:

1. Layer the ingredients in the following sequence in a transparent glass or bowl:
2. As a basis, start with a tablespoon of Greek yogurt.
3. Top with a layer of strawberry slices.
4. Add another layer of Greek yogurt after that.
5. Spread some blueberries on top.
6. Drizzle with maple syrup or honey.
7. Spread Greek yogurt over another layer.

8. Spread some raspberries on top.

9. Add chopped nuts and granola to the parfait's top.

10. Serve right away and savor the complex, colorful flavors.

Nutritional Information (per serving):

- Calories: 250

- Protein: 12g

- Fat: 6g

- Carbohydrates: 40g

- Fiber: 6g

Difficulty: Easy

This vibrant and wholesome parfait offers a good mix of antioxidant-rich berries, protein from Greek yogurt, and fiber-rich granola. This easy yet delicious breakfast is full of fiber, vitamins, and minerals and is a great way to start the day. Because of its low difficulty level, children can construct it with little help.

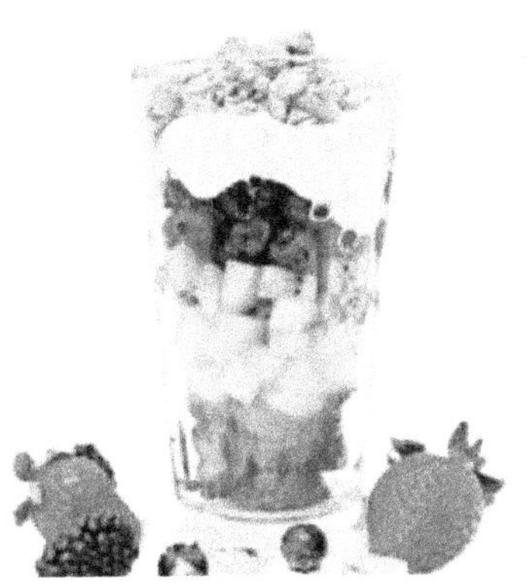

Wholesome Whole Grain Pancakes

Ingredients:

- Whole grain pancake mix (1 cup)
- Mixed fresh berries (sliced strawberries, blueberries, raspberries) (1 cup)
- Greek yogurt or honey for topping (optional)
- Cooking spray or butter for greasing the pan

Instructions:

1. As directed on the box, prepare the whole-grain pancake batter.
2. Grease a non-stick pan or griddle with cooking spray or butter and heat it over medium heat.

3. Using roughly 1/4 cup of batter for each pancake, pour pancake batter onto the pan to create little pancakes.

4. As each pancake cooks, scatter a handful of mixed fresh berries over it.

5. Cook the pancake until bubbles appear on its surface, then turn it over and continue cooking until the second side is golden brown.

6. Continue until the batter is all utilized.

7. Top the pancakes with more fresh berries and, if preferred, a drizzle of honey or a dollop of Greek yogurt.

Nutritional Information (per serving):

- Calories: 200
- Protein: 7g
- Fat: 2g
- Carbohydrates: 40g
- Fiber: 5g

Difficulty: Moderate

A healthier take on a beloved breakfast dish, these whole-grain pancakes are delicious. They provide a well-rounded breakfast choice since they are full of fiber from whole grains and a quick hit of antioxidants from fresh berries. Because of the cooking process, the difficulty level is moderate, so children who have some culinary experience or adult supervision may find it appropriate.

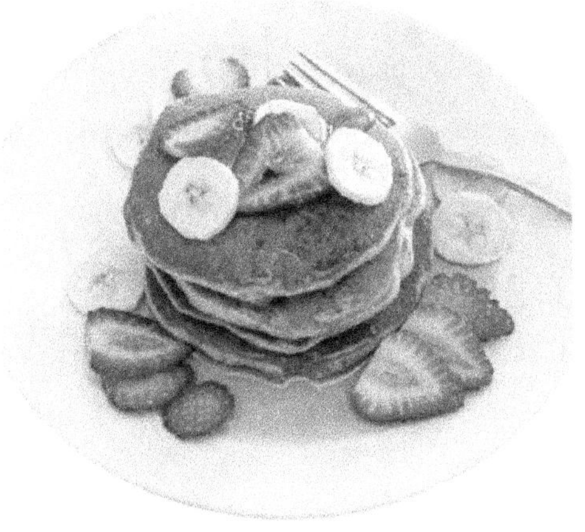

Veggie-Packed Frittata Bites

Ingredients:

- Eggs (4 large)
- Bell peppers (diced) (1/2 cup)
- Spinach (chopped) (1 cup)
- Cherry tomatoes (halved) (1/2 cup)
- Feta cheese (crumbled) (1/4 cup)
- Olive oil (1 tablespoon)
- Salt and pepper to taste
- Fresh herbs (parsley, basil) for garnish (optional)

Instructions:

1. Set the oven's temperature to 175°C/350°F.
2. Beat the eggs and add the salt and pepper in a mixing bowl.
3. In an oven-safe skillet, warm the olive oil over medium heat.
4. Add the chopped spinach and cherry tomatoes after sautéing the diced bell peppers until they start to soften. Cook until spinach starts to wilt.

5. Evenly cover the vegetables in the skillet with the beaten eggs.

6. Top with feta cheese crumbles.

7. Cook over medium heat for 2 to 3 minutes, or until the edges begin to firm.

8. After transferring the pan to the oven, warm it and bake for 10 to 12 minutes, or until the frittata is cooked through and has a hint of color.

9. Take it out of the oven and give it some time to cool. Next, cut the frittata into triangles or squares that are bite-sized.

10. If desired, garnish with fresh herbs.

11. Heat or serve at room temperature.

Nutritional Information (per serving):

- Calories: 120
- Protein: 9g
- Fat: 8g
- Carbohydrates: 4g
- Fiber: 1g

Difficulty: Intermediate

These colorful veggie-packed frittata bites are a great way to get your fill of vitamins and minerals. Although this breakfast choice, which is high in protein, is reasonably simple to make, using the oven and cooktop may need adult supervision.

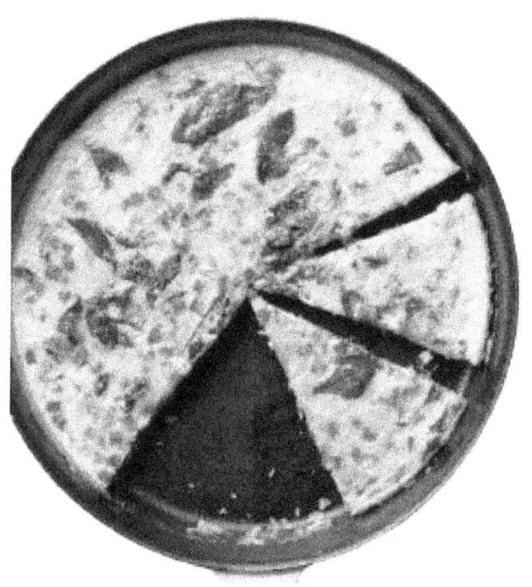

Mediterranean Veggie Omelette

Ingredients:

- Eggs (2 large)
- Chopped Mediterranean vegetables (zucchini, red onion, cherry tomatoes) (1 cup)
- Crumbled feta cheese or goat cheese (2 tablespoons)
- Fresh herbs (parsley, basil) (1 tablespoon, chopped)

- Olive oil (1 tablespoon)
- Salt and pepper to taste

Instructions:

1. In a nonstick skillet, warm the olive oil over medium heat.
2. When the vegetables are soft but still somewhat crunchy, add the chopped Mediterranean veggies to the pan and sauté them.
3. Beat the eggs and add salt and pepper to taste in a bowl.
4. Evenly cover the skillet's sautéed veggies with the beaten eggs.
5. After letting the eggs set a little on the edges, carefully raise the edges with a spatula to allow the raw eggs to fall to the bottom.
6. Sprinkle equally over one side of the omelet (when it's nearly finished but still somewhat runny on top), feta, or goat cheese crumbles.
7. Gently fold the remaining omelet half over the side with the cheese.
8. To melt the cheese and finish frying the eggs, heat for one additional minute.

9. The omelet should slide onto a platter.

10. Add freshly chopped herbs as a garnish.

Nutritional Information (per serving):

- Calories: 180

- Protein: 12g

- Fat: 12g

- Carbohydrates: 6g

- Fiber: 2g

Difficulty: Easy

Packed with healthy veggies and egg protein, this Mediterranean Veggie Omelette is sure to satisfy your appetite. It's an easy breakfast choice that tastes well and is simple enough for youngsters to make with minimal culinary abilities.

Berry Blast Smoothie Bowl

Ingredients:

- Greek yogurt or almond milk (1 cup)

- Mixed frozen berries (strawberries, blueberries, raspberries) (1 cup)

- Banana (1, sliced)
- Toppings: Granola (1/4 cup), sliced almonds (2 tablespoons), shredded coconut (2 tablespoons), fresh fruit for garnish

Instructions:

1. Sliced banana, mixed frozen berries, and almond milk or Greek yogurt should all be combined in a blender.
2. Blend till creamy and smooth. If necessary, add a little more liquid to the smoothie to make it thicker.
3. Transfer the blended drink to a bowl.
4. Sprinkle granola, chopped almonds, shredded coconut, and fresh fruit pieces on top of the smoothie bowl as decoration.

Nutritional Information (per serving):

- Calories: 280
- Protein: 10g
- Fat: 8g
- Carbohydrates: 45g
- Fiber: 8g

Difficulty: Easy

A healthy and hydrating breakfast choice, this Berry Blast Smoothie Bowl is high in fiber, vitamins, and antioxidants. It's a fun breakfast option that kids can put together on their own with little effort since it's simple to make and adaptable with different toppings.

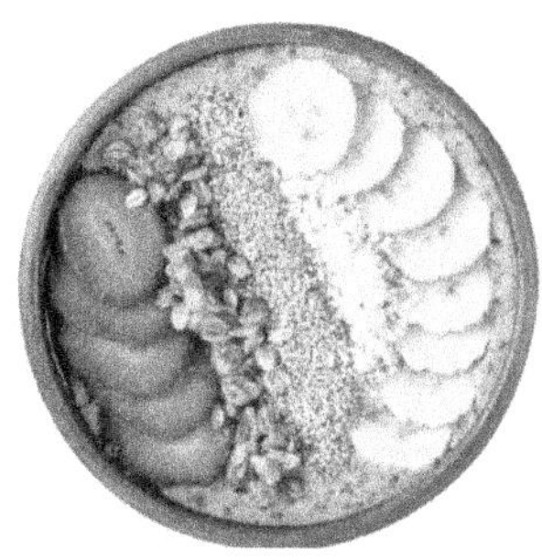

Mediterranean Veggie Hummus Wraps

Ingredients:

- Whole grain wraps or tortillas (4)
- Hummus (1 cup)
- Cherry tomatoes (sliced) (1 cup)
- Cucumber (sliced) (1 cup)
- Red bell pepper (thinly sliced) (1 cup)
- Red onion (thinly sliced) (1/2 cup)
- Baby spinach or mixed greens (2 cups)
- Kalamata olives (sliced) (1/4 cup)
- Feta cheese (crumbled) (1/4 cup)
- Olive oil (2 tablespoons)
- Balsamic vinegar (1 tablespoon)
- Salt and pepper to taste

Instructions:

1. Arrange the tortillas or whole grain wraps in a flat layer.
2. Each wrap should have a thick coating of hummus on it, with a thin border all the way around.

3. Arrange the feta cheese crumbles, sliced Kalamata olives, baby spinach or mixed greens, cucumber, red bell pepper, red onion, and cherry tomatoes in a layer on top of the hummus.

4. Over the vegetables, drizzle some olive oil and balsamic vinegar.

5. To taste, add salt and pepper for seasoning.

6. To make a tight wrap, carefully roll up each wrap, tucking in the edges as you go.

7. To serve, cut each wrap in half or smaller pieces using a diagonal cut.

Nutritional Information (per serving - 1 wrap):

- Calories: 280
- Protein: 9g
- Fat: 12g
- Carbohydrates: 35g
- Fiber: 8g

Difficulty: Easy

The protein-rich hummus, nutritious grains, and a well-balanced combination of veggies are all present in these Mediterranean Veggie Hummus Wraps. They provide a tasty, wholesome snack alternative and are simple to put together. Because of its low difficulty level, children can prepare it with some help.

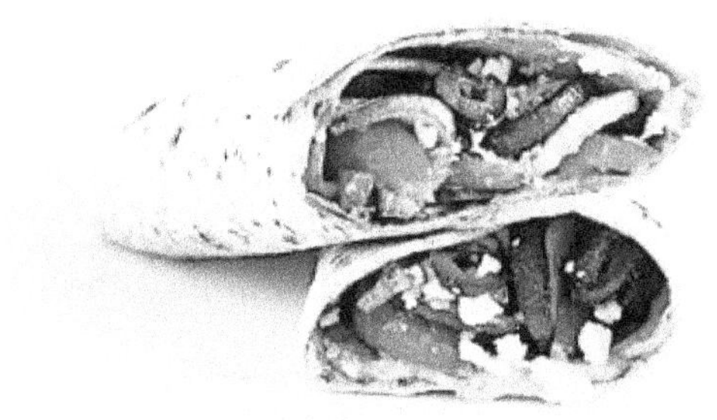

Fruit and Nut Energy Balls

Ingredients:

- Medjool dates (pitted) (1 cup)

- Almonds (1/2 cup)

- Walnuts (1/2 cup)

- Dried apricots (1/2 cup)

- Dried cranberries (1/4 cup)

- Unsweetened shredded coconut (1/4 cup)

- Chia seeds (2 tablespoons)

- Honey or maple syrup (2 tablespoons)

- Vanilla extract (1 teaspoon)

- Optional: Cocoa powder or cinnamon for coating

Instructions:

1. Pitted dates, almonds, walnuts, dried cranberries, dried apricots, chia seeds, shredded coconut, honey or maple syrup, and vanilla essence should all be combined in a food processor.
2. Pulse the ingredients until a homogenous, sticky substance forms that presses together.
3. Take small spoonfuls of the mixture and roll them between your hands into tiny balls about the size of an inch.
4. You may add more taste by rolling the energy balls in cinnamon or chocolate powder if you'd like.
5. To set, put the energy balls on a tray lined with parchment paper and chill for at least half an hour.

Nutritional Information (per serving - 2 energy balls):

- Calories: 180
- Protein: 4g
- Fat: 9g
- Carbohydrates: 24g
- Fiber: 4g

Difficulty: Easy

Fruit and Nut Energy Balls are a delicious snack that combines the health of nuts and seeds with the natural sweetness of dates and dried fruits. They are a great on-the-go snack or a fast energy boost for busy youngsters since they are simple to make and provide a rush of energy. Because of the simple difficulty level, children may participate in the preparation with little adult supervision.

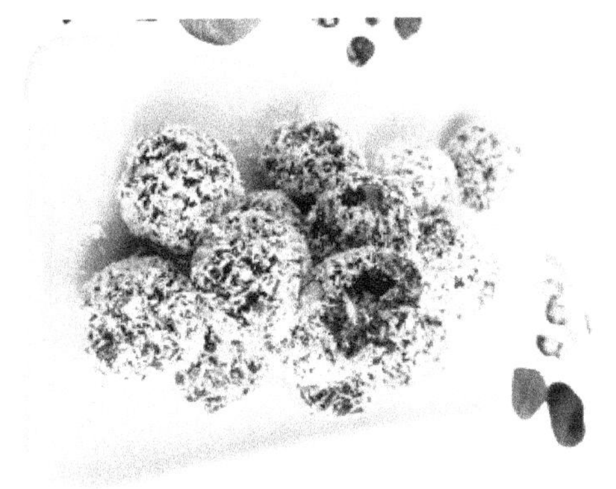

Greek Yogurt Parfait Cups with Granola

Ingredients:

- Greek yogurt (2 cups)
- Mixed fresh berries (strawberries, blueberries, raspberries) (1 cup)

- Honey or maple syrup (2 tablespoons)

- Granola (1/2 cup)

- Optional: Sliced almonds or chopped nuts for topping

Instructions:

1. Combine the Greek yogurt and maple syrup in a mixing dish and stir until well-mixed.

2. Clean and prep the assortment of fresh berries.

3. Alternately arrange the Greek yogurt mixture, mixed fresh berries, and granola in small cups or bowls.

4. Once the cups are full, continue layering until a layer of granola is on top.

5. Optionally top the granola layer with chopped or sliced almonds.

6. Before serving, place the parfait glasses in the refrigerator for at least 15 to 20 minutes to enable the flavors to mingle and the granola to get a little softer.

Nutritional Information (per serving):

- Calories: 220

- Protein: 14g

- Fat: 6g

- Carbohydrates: 30g

- Fiber: 4g

Difficulty: Easy

The delicious combination of creamy Greek yogurt, sweet mixed berries, and crispy granola is present in these Greek Yogurt Parfait Cups with Granola. They provide a well-balanced snack that is high in fiber, protein, and antioxidants, and they are easy to put together. Because of its low difficulty level, children may take part in the preparation process.

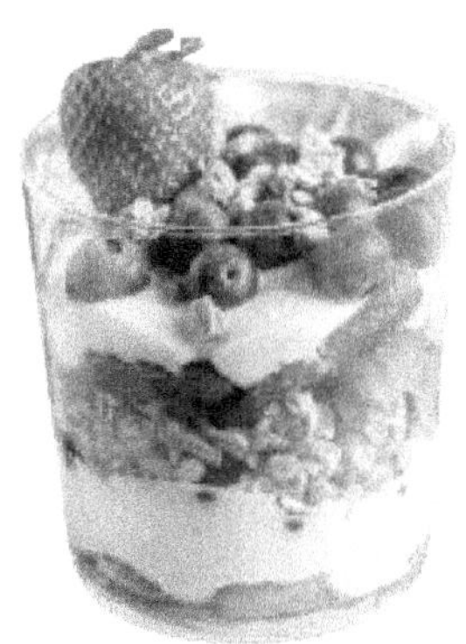

Fresh Fruit Popsicles

Ingredients:

- Assorted fresh fruits (strawberries, kiwi, blueberries, mango, etc.)
- Fruit juice or coconut water
- Honey or agave syrup (optional, for added sweetness)

Instructions:

1. The fresh fruits should be cleaned and then cut into bite-sized pieces.
2. Evenly divide the fruit pieces among the Popsicle molds, alternating between various fruits in each mold to provide color and variation.
3. Cover the fruit pieces in the molds with fruit juice or coconut water. For added sweetness, feel free to use a tiny quantity of honey or agave syrup.
4. Place a Popsicle stick into every mold.
5. After putting the Popsicle molds in the freezer, leave them there for at least four to six hours, or until they are fully frozen.
6. To remove the popsicles with ease once they have frozen, briefly submerge the molds in warm water.

Nutritional Information (per serving - 1 Popsicle):

Nutritional values may vary depending on the fruits and liquids used.

Difficulty: Easy

Simple to make and a fantastic hands-on activity for kids with adult supervision, these Fresh Fruit Popsicles are a fun and simple way for kids to enjoy fresh fruits while remaining cool. They're adaptable to other fruits and liquids.

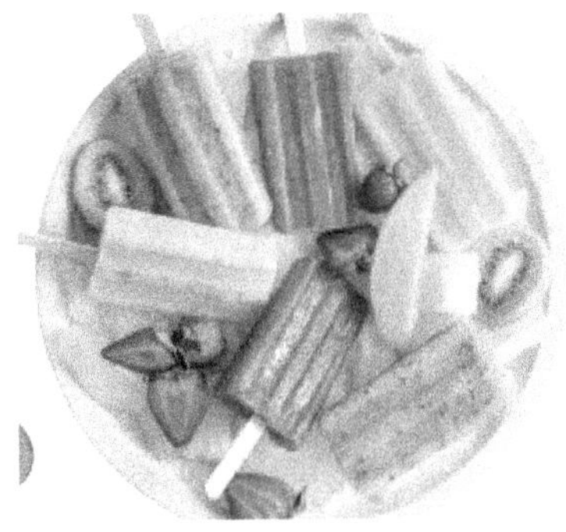

Greek Yogurt Berry Bark

Ingredients:

- Greek yogurt (2 cups)
- Mixed fresh berries (strawberries, blueberries, raspberries) (1 cup)
- Honey or maple syrup (2 tablespoons)

- Optional: Chopped nuts (almonds, walnuts) or shredded coconut for topping

Instructions:

1. Use parchment paper to line a baking sheet.
2. Blend the Greek yogurt with honey or maple syrup in a bowl until its smooth.
3. Create a thin layer of the Greek yogurt mixture on the baking sheet that has been prepared.
4. Gently press the mixed fresh berries into the yogurt layer by scattering them over it.
5. For extra taste and texture, sprinkle with shredded coconut or chopped almonds.
6. The baking sheet should be frozen for at least two to three hours, or until it is set.
7. Using a knife or your hands, cut the yogurt bark into smaller pieces once it has frozen.

Nutritional Information (per serving):

Nutritional values may vary depending on the specific ingredients used.

Difficulty: Easy

This Greek Yogurt Berry Bark combines the natural sweetness of fresh berries with the creamy texture of Greek yogurt, making it a pleasant and healthful snack alternative. It provides an equilibrium of antioxidants, vitamins, and protein. Because it's easy to make, even youngsters can assist in creating this fun and easy meal.

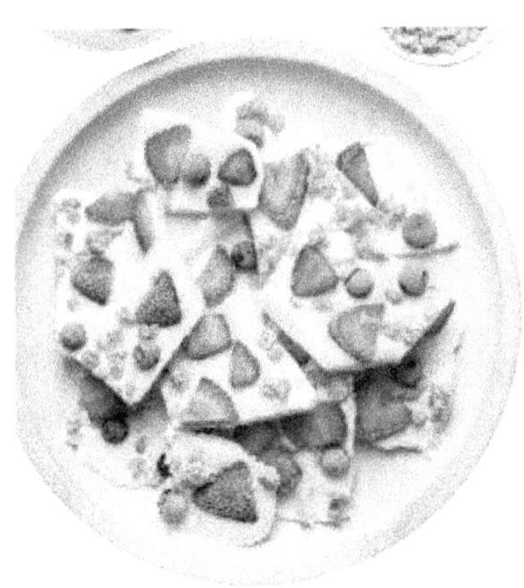

Mediterranean Veggie and Hummus Wraps

Ingredients:

- Whole grain wraps or tortillas (4)
- Hummus (1 cup)
- Cherry tomatoes (sliced) (1 cup)
- Cucumber (sliced) (1 cup)
- Red bell pepper (thinly sliced) (1 cup)
- Red onion (thinly sliced) (1/2 cup)
- Baby spinach or mixed greens (2 cups)
- Kalamata olives (sliced) (1/4 cup)
- Feta cheese (crumbled) (1/4 cup)
- Olive oil (2 tablespoons)
- Balsamic vinegar (1 tablespoon)
- Salt and pepper to taste

Instructions:

1. Arrange the tortillas or whole grain wraps in a flat layer.

2. Each wrap should have a thick coating of hummus on it, with a thin border all the way around.

3. Arrange the feta cheese crumbles, sliced Kalamata olives, baby spinach or mixed greens, cucumber, red bell pepper, red onion, and cherry tomatoes in a layer on top of the hummus.

4. Over the vegetables, drizzle some olive oil and balsamic vinegar.

5. To taste, add salt and pepper for seasoning.

6. To make a tight wrap, carefully roll up each wrap, tucking in the edges as you go.

7. To serve, cut each wrap in half or smaller pieces using a diagonal cut.

Nutritional Information (per serving - 1 wrap):

- Calories: 300
- Protein: 10g
- Fat: 12g
- Carbohydrates: 40g
- Fiber: 7g

Difficulty: Easy

These colorful, tasty, and nutrient-dense Mediterranean Veggie and hummus Wraps are a great lunch choice. With their abundance of fresh veggies, high-protein hummus, and whole-grain wraps, they provide a well-balanced lunch that is appropriate for children. Because of its low complexity level, this dish is perfect for youngsters to help prepare with minor guidance.

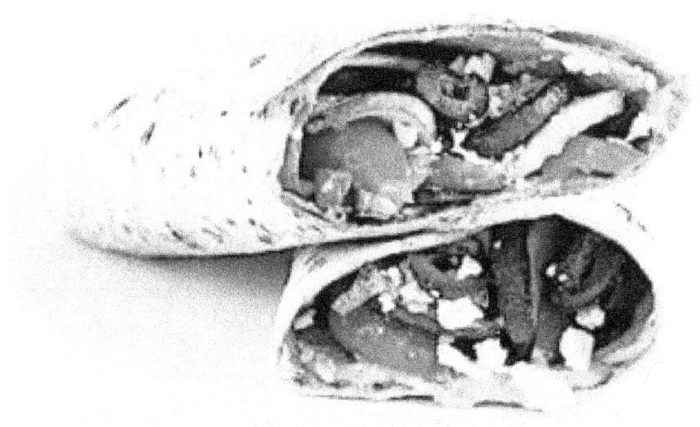

Greek Chicken Souvlaki with Tzatziki Sauce

Ingredients:

For Chicken Souvlaki:

- Boneless, skinless chicken breasts or thighs (1 pound, cut into cubes)

- Olive oil (3 tablespoons)

- Lemon juice (2 tablespoons)

- Garlic cloves (minced) (2 cloves)

- Dried oregano (1 teaspoon)

- Salt and pepper to taste

- Skewers (if using wooden skewers, soak them in water for 30 minutes before use)

For Tzatziki Sauce:

- Greek yogurt (1 cup)

- Cucumber (peeled, seeded, grated) (1/2 cup)

- Garlic clove (minced) (1 clove)

- Lemon juice (1 tablespoon)

- Fresh dill (chopped) (1 tablespoon)

- Salt and pepper to taste

Instructions:

For Chicken Souvlaki:

1. Olive oil, lemon juice, dried oregano, minced garlic, salt, and pepper should all be combined in a bowl.

2. Coat well after adding the cubed chicken to the marinade. Let it marinate for a minimum of half an hour in the fridge.

3. After marinating, thread the chicken onto skewers.

4. On a prepared grill or grill pan, cook the chicken skewers over medium-high heat, flipping them regularly, until they are cooked through, 8 to 10 minutes.

For Tzatziki Sauce:

1. Greek yogurt, grated cucumber, minced garlic, lemon juice, chopped dill, salt, and pepper should all be combined in a different bowl.

2. Mix well to blend. Store in the fridge until needed.

3. Present the handmade tzatziki sauce beside the grilled chicken souvlaki.

Nutritional Information (per serving):

Nutritional values may vary based on portion size and specific ingredients used.

Difficulty: Intermediate

This Tzatziki Sauced Greek Chicken Souvlaki is a tasty and filling lunch dish. Although it requires marinating and grilling, the preparation is simple, so youngsters with some culinary expertise or adult supervision may make this meal easily.

Quinoa and Chickpea Greek Salad

Ingredients:

For the Salad:

- Cooked quinoa (2 cups)
- Chickpeas (1 can, drained and rinsed)
- Cucumber (diced) (1 cup)
- Cherry tomatoes (halved) (1 cup)
- Red onion (finely chopped) (1/2 cup)
- Kalamata olives (pitted and sliced) (1/4 cup)
- Feta cheese (crumbled) (1/2 cup)
- Fresh parsley (chopped) (1/4 cup)

For the Dressing:

- Extra-virgin olive oil (1/4 cup)
- Red wine vinegar (2 tablespoons)
- Lemon juice (1 tablespoon)

- Dried oregano (1 teaspoon)
- Salt and pepper to taste

Instructions:

1. The cooked quinoa, drained chickpeas, diced cucumber, halved cherry tomatoes, finely chopped red onion, sliced Kalamata olives, crumbled feta cheese, and chopped fresh parsley should all be combined in a large mixing dish.
2. To create the dressing, combine the lemon juice, extra virgin olive oil, red wine vinegar, dried oregano, salt, and pepper in a small bowl.
3. Over the quinoa and chickpea mixture, drizzle the dressing. To evenly coat all ingredients, lightly toss.
4. If necessary, taste and adjust the seasoning.
5. To enable the flavors to mingle, chill the salad in the fridge for at least half an hour before serving.
6. If preferred, serve as an accompaniment to grilled chicken or fish or as the main course.

Nutritional Information (per serving):

Nutritional values may vary based on portion size and specific ingredients used.

Difficulty: Easy

This tasty and healthful lunch choice, loaded with fiber, protein, and taste, is a quinoa and chickpea salad. The dish offers a great flavor of the Mediterranean diet and is very easy to create. Children may help with preparation as long as an adult is supervising them.

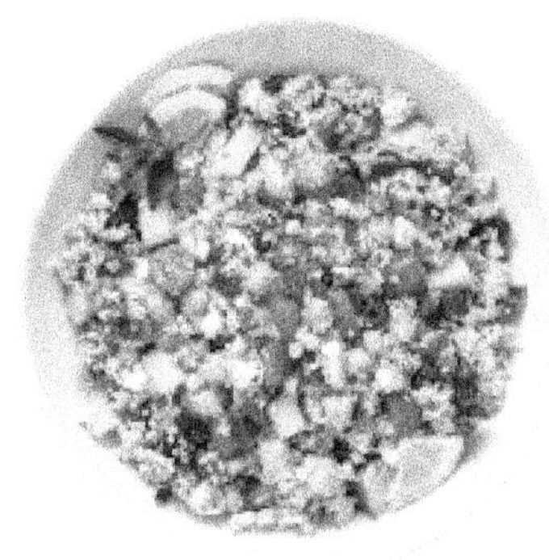

Lemon-Herb Baked Fish

Ingredients:

- White fish fillets (such as cod, tilapia, or halibut) (4 fillets)
- Olive oil (2 tablespoons)
- Lemon juice (2 tablespoons)
- Garlic cloves (minced) (2 cloves)

- Fresh herbs (such as parsley, dill, or thyme) (2 tablespoons, chopped)
- Lemon zest (from 1 lemon)
- Salt and pepper to taste
- Lemon slices (for garnish)

Instructions:

1. Turn the oven on to 375°F, or 190°C. Use olive oil to grease or line a baking dish with parchment paper.
2. To make a marinade, combine olive oil, lemon juice, minced garlic, chopped fresh herbs, lemon zest, salt, and pepper in a small bowl.
3. Using paper towels, pat dry the fish fillets and transfer them to the baking dish that has been prepared.
4. Make sure the fish fillets are uniformly covered by pouring the marinade over them. Alternatively, you may brush the marinade onto the fillets.
5. Top each fillet with a slice of lemon for taste.
6. Fish should be baked for 12 to 15 minutes in a preheated oven, or until it is cooked through and flake readily with a fork.

7. Take it out of the oven and let it a few minutes to settle before serving.

8. For a full and healthy supper, serve the lemon-herb baked fish with quinoa or a side salad.

Nutritional Information (per serving):

Nutritional values may vary based on the type and size of fish used.

Difficulty: Easy

This recipe for Lemon-Herb Baked Fish is straightforward, tasty, and simple to make. Kids may actively engage in the cooking process under adult supervision, and it's a nutritious and protein-rich lunch choice.

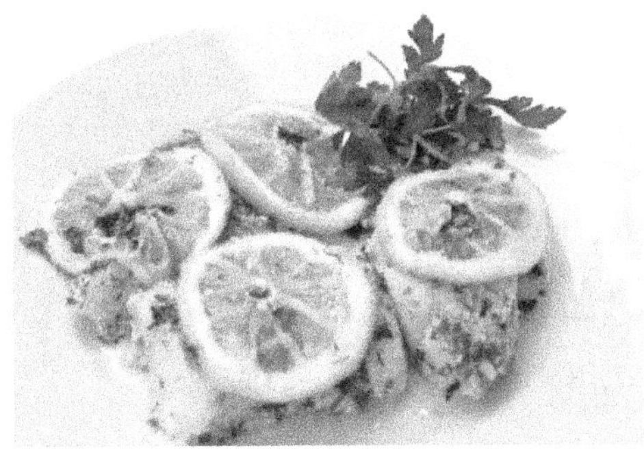

Mediterranean Veggie Pita Pockets

Ingredients:

- Whole wheat pita bread (4 rounds)
- Hummus (1 cup)
- Cherry tomatoes (halved) (1 cup)
- Cucumber (diced) (1 cup)
- Red bell pepper (thinly sliced) (1 cup)
- Red onion (thinly sliced) (1/2 cup)
- Kalamata olives (pitted and sliced) (1/4 cup)
- Feta cheese (crumbled) (1/4 cup)
- Olive oil (2 tablespoons)
- Balsamic vinegar (1 tablespoon)
- Fresh parsley (chopped) (2 tablespoons)
- Salt and pepper to taste

Instructions:

1. To create pockets, cut the whole wheat pita rounds in half. Carefully open every pocket to provide room for filling.
2. Put a good dollop of hummus into each pita pocket.

3. Cherry tomatoes, diced cucumber, red bell pepper, red onion, sliced Kalamata olives, crumbled feta cheese, and chopped fresh parsley should all be combined in a dish.

4. Pour balsamic vinegar and olive oil over the vegetable mixture. To taste, add salt and pepper for seasoning. To mix, toss.

5. Divide the prepared vegetable mixture equally among the pita pockets and stuff them with it.

6. Serve the tasty and wholesome Mediterranean Veggie Pita Pockets for lunch.

Nutritional Information (per serving):

Nutritional values may vary based on specific ingredients and quantities used.

Difficulty: Easy

With their abundance of fresh veggies, zesty spices, and creamy hummus, these Mediterranean Veggie Pita Pockets make a filling and nutritious supper. They provide a fun lunch alternative since they are simple to put together and, with little supervision, kids may enjoy forming their own pita pockets.

Mediterranean Veggie and Chickpea Stew

Ingredients:

- Olive oil (2 tablespoons)
- Onion (diced) (1 large)
- Garlic cloves (minced) (3 cloves)
- Carrots (sliced) (2 medium)
- Red bell pepper (diced) (1)
- Zucchini (sliced) (1)
- Eggplant (diced) (1)
- Canned diced tomatoes (14 oz)
- Vegetable broth (2 cups)
- Chickpeas (cooked or canned, drained and rinsed) (1 can)
- Dried oregano (1 teaspoon)
- Dried basil (1 teaspoon)
- Dried thyme (1/2 teaspoon)
- Salt and pepper to taste
- Fresh parsley (chopped, for garnish)

Instructions:

1. Heat the olive oil in a big saucepan or Dutch oven over medium heat.

2. Add minced garlic and chopped onion. The onion should be sautéed until transparent.

3. Toss in the chopped eggplant, diced red bell pepper, sliced zucchini, and sliced carrots. Simmer the veggies for a few minutes, or until they begin to become tender.

4. Add the veggie broth and diced tomatoes from a can. Mix everything.

5. Toss in the canned or cooked chickpeas, salt, pepper, dried thyme, dried basil, and dried oregano. Mix thoroughly.

6. After bringing the stew to a boil, turn down the heat. Once the flavors are well combined and the veggies are soft, cover and simmer for 20 to 25 minutes.

7. Before serving, adjust the spice as necessary and top with freshly chopped parsley.

Nutritional Information (per serving): Nutritional values may vary based on specific ingredients and servings.

Difficulty: Easy

Rich in plant-based protein and veggies, this Mediterranean Veggie and Chickpea Stew is a filling and healthy supper choice. It's easy to make, and kids may help cook it as long as they are supervised. It is a tasty and adaptable dinner that can be customized to suit individual tastes.

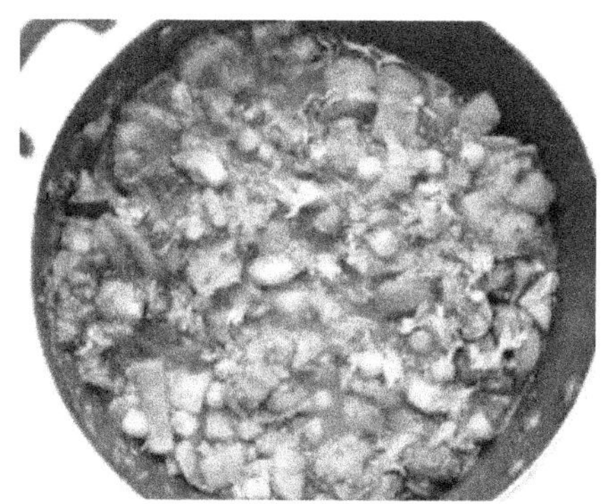

Lemony Garlic Shrimp with Quinoa

Ingredients:

- Shrimp (peeled and deveined) (1 pound)
- Quinoa (1 cup, rinsed)
- Olive oil (2 tablespoons)
- Garlic cloves (minced) (3 cloves)
- Lemon zest (from 1 lemon)
- Lemon juice (from 1 lemon)

- Cherry tomatoes (halved) (1 cup)

- Baby spinach (2 cups)

- Fresh parsley (chopped) (2 tablespoons)

- Salt and pepper to taste

Instructions:

1. Follow the directions on the box to cook the quinoa. After cooking, put it aside.

2. Add the minced garlic, lemon zest, lemon juice, olive oil, salt, and pepper to a bowl and marinate the shrimp. Give it 10 to 15 minutes to sit.

3. Add a little amount of olive oil to a skillet or pan and heat it to medium. The marinated shrimp should be grilled for two to three minutes on each side, or until they are pink and fully cooked. After taking the shrimp out of the pan, put it aside.

4. If necessary, add a little more olive oil to the same pan. Cherry tomatoes cut in half should be sautéed till tender.

5. Cook the young spinach in the pan until it wilts.

6. Toss everything together for a minute or two to blend and reheat the cooked shrimp, then return them to the pan.

7. Arrange the cooked quinoa atop a bed of lemony garlic shrimp.

8. Before serving, sprinkle some freshly chopped parsley on top.

Nutritional Information (per serving):

Nutritional values may vary based on specific ingredients and servings.

Difficulty: Easy

For supper, try this tasty and protein-rich lemony garlic shrimp with quinoa. It's easy to make and has a delicious blend of spicy tastes. Under adult supervision, children may help with duties like measuring, stirring, or prepping the shrimp.

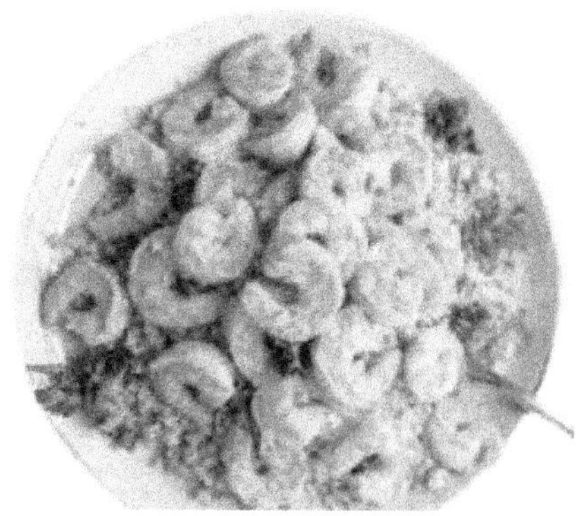

Mediterranean Baked Chicken with Herbs

Ingredients:

- Chicken thighs or breasts (4 pieces)
- Olive oil (3 tablespoons)
- Lemon juice (from 1 lemon)
- Garlic cloves (minced) (3 cloves)
- Dried oregano (1 teaspoon)
- Dried basil (1 teaspoon)
- Dried thyme (1/2 teaspoon)
- Paprika (1 teaspoon)
- Salt and pepper to taste
- Lemon slices for garnish (optional)
- Fresh parsley (chopped, for garnish)

Instructions:

1. Turn the oven on to 375°F, or 190°C. Lightly coat a baking dish with olive oil.
2. To make a marinade, combine olive oil, lemon juice, minced garlic, dried thyme, dried basil, dried oregano, paprika, salt, and pepper in a bowl.

3. After using paper towels to pat dry, transfer the chicken pieces to the ready baking dish.

4. Make sure the chicken pieces are well covered by pouring the marinade over them. Work the marinade into the chicken with your hands.

5. For extra taste (optional), arrange lemon slices on top of the chicken pieces.

6. Bake for 25 to 30 minutes, or until the chicken is cooked through and the juices are clear, in a preheated oven.

7. After cooking, take the chicken out of the oven and give it some time to rest.

8. Before serving, scatter some freshly cut parsley over the chicken.

9. Nutritional Data (per serving): Depending on the components and serving sizes, different nutritional values may apply.

Nutritional Information (per serving):

Nutritional values may vary based on specific ingredients and servings.

Difficulty: Easy

Simple and tasty, this Mediterranean Baked Chicken with Herbs meal brings out the taste of the region's fragrant herbs. Because it's simple to make, kids may assist with activities like combining the marinade or placing the chicken in the baking dish as long as an adult is watching.

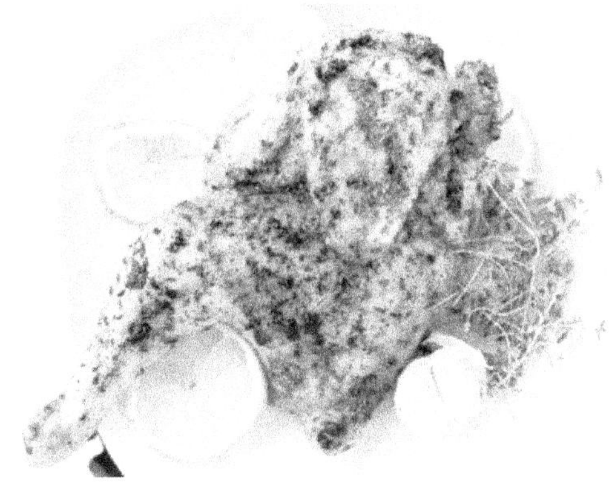

Greek-Style Grilled Lamb Kebabs

Ingredients:

- Lamb leg or shoulder (1 pound, cubed)
- Red onion (cut into chunks) (1)
- Red bell pepper (cut into chunks) (1)
- Cherry tomatoes (1 cup)
- Olive oil (1/4 cup)
- Lemon juice (from 1 lemon)

- Garlic cloves (minced) (3 cloves)

- Fresh oregano (chopped) (2 tablespoons)

- Salt and pepper to taste

- Metal or wooden skewers (if using wooden skewers, soak them in water for 30 minutes before use)

Instructions:

1. To avoid burning, soak wooden skewers in water for at least half an hour before using them.

2. Make a marinade in a bowl by combining olive oil, lemon juice, minced garlic, chopped fresh oregano, salt, and pepper.

3. Transfer the cubed lamb to a shallow dish and cover it with the marinade. Coat the lamb evenly by tossing it. For optimal taste, marinate in the fridge for at least one to two hours, preferably overnight.

4. Set the grill's temperature to medium-high.

5. On skewers, thread marinated lamb cubes in alternate rows with cherry tomatoes, red onion, and red bell pepper pieces.

6. Turn the kebabs every few minutes while grilling them for approximately 10 to 12 minutes, or until the

lamb is cooked through and the veggies have a hint of sear.

7. Before serving, take the kebabs from the grill and give them some time to rest.

8. Serve the grilled lamb kebabs in the Greek manner with pita bread, tzatziki sauce, or Greek salad on the side.

Nutritional Information (per serving):

Nutritional values may vary based on specific ingredients and servings.

Difficulty: Intermediate

These fragrant and savory Greek-style grilled Lamb Kebabs are the ideal meal for a supper with a Mediterranean flair. Kids may help thread the skewers or prepare the marinade while an adult supervises them throughout the marinating and grilling phases of the preparation.

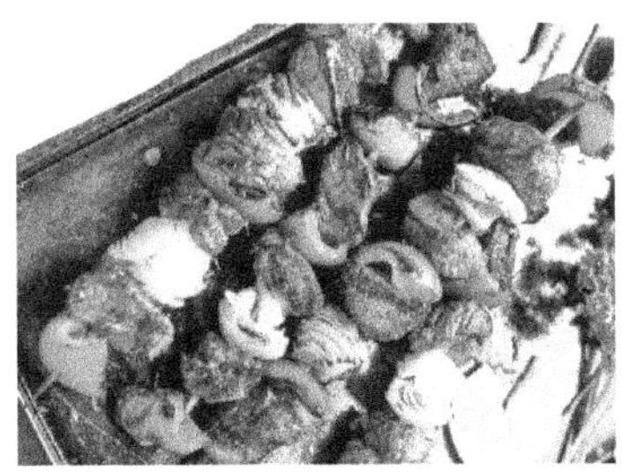

Mediterranean-style Stuffed Bell Peppers

Ingredients:

- Bell peppers (4 large, any color)
- Ground lamb or beef (1 pound)
- Olive oil (2 tablespoons)
- Onion (diced) (1)
- Garlic cloves (minced) (3 cloves)
- Tomatoes (diced) (2 medium)
- Cooked quinoa or rice (1 cup)
- Kalamata olives (pitted and chopped) (1/4 cup)
- Feta cheese (crumbled) (1/2 cup)
- Fresh parsley (chopped) (2 tablespoons)
- Dried oregano (1 teaspoon)
- Salt and pepper to taste
- Tomato sauce or marinara sauce (1 cup)
- Grated mozzarella cheese (optional, for topping)

Instructions:

1. Turn the oven on to 375°F, or 190°C. Lightly coat a baking dish with olive oil.

2. Remove the bell peppers' seeds and membranes by cutting off the tops. Give the peppers a good rinse.

3. Heat the olive oil in a pan over medium heat. Add the minced garlic and onion and sauté until the ingredients are tender.

4. Cook the ground beef or lamb in the pan until it becomes brown. If necessary, drain the extra fat.

5. Add chopped fresh parsley, dried oregano, salt, pepper, chopped Kalamata olives, cooked quinoa or rice, and diced tomatoes. Simmer for a few minutes, or until well cooked and well blended.

6. Tightly stuff the cooked beef and rice/quinoa mixture into each bell pepper.

7. In the baking dish that has been prepared, place the filled bell peppers upright.

8. Cover the filled peppers with a layer of marinara or tomato sauce.

9. Bake the peppers for 35 to 40 minutes, or until they are soft while covering the oven dish with foil.

10. Take off the foil if you'd like, cover the peppers with shredded mozzarella cheese, and bake for a further

five minutes, or until the cheese melts and becomes brown.

11. Before serving, take the filled bell peppers out of the oven and allow them to cool for a few minutes.

Nutritional Information (per serving):

Nutritional values may vary based on specific ingredients and servings.

Difficulty: Intermediate

This dish of Mediterranean-style stuffed Bell Peppers is filling and delicious. Even though there may be many phases in the preparation, children may assist with adult supervision while stuffing peppers or combining filling.

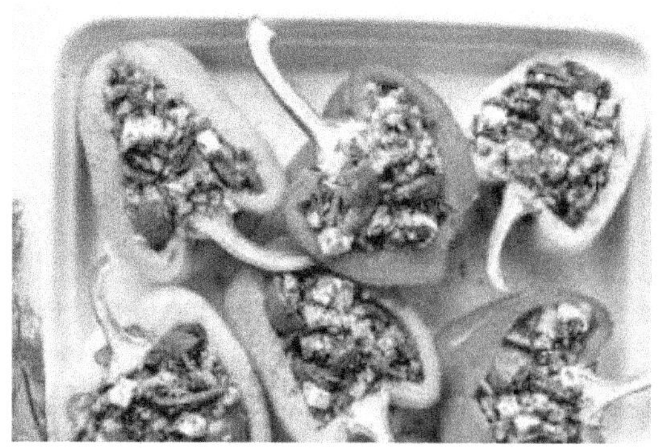

CHAPTER 6: SWEET TREATS AND DESSERTS

Greek Yogurt Frozen Fruit Pops

Ingredients:

- Greek yogurt (2 cups)
- Mixed fresh berries (strawberries, blueberries, raspberries) (1 cup)
- Honey or maple syrup (2 tablespoons)
- Optional: Sliced almonds or chopped nuts for topping

Instructions:

1. Smoothly incorporate Greek yogurt, mixed fresh berries, and honey or maple syrup in a food processor or blender.
2. Leaving a little amount of room at the top for expansion, pour the mixture into the Popsicle molds.
3. Stick Popsicles into the molds.
4. Optional: For extra texture, top each pop with sliced or chopped almonds.

5. The Popsicle molds should be frozen for at least four to six hours, or until they are totally solid.

6. To remove the popsicles with ease once they have frozen, briefly submerge the molds in warm water.

Nutritional Information (per serving - 1 Popsicle):

Nutritional values may vary based on the specific ingredients used.

Difficulty: Easy

In place of store-bought popsicles, try these delicious and nutritious Greek Yogurt Frozen Fruit Pops. Brimming with the freshness of fresh fruit and Greek yogurt, they provide a cool, wholesome dessert option for children. Because of its low complexity level, children may help prepare this easy meal with adult supervision. It's also a fun and straightforward recipe.

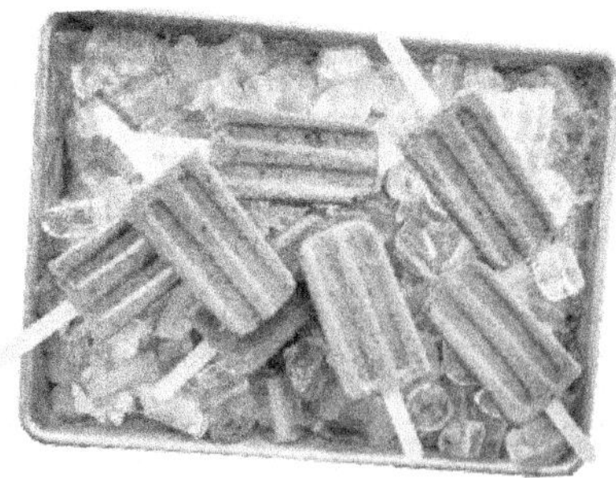

Honey and Yogurt Parfait with Fresh Berries

Ingredients:

- Greek yogurt (2 cups)
- Honey (2 tablespoons)
- Mixed fresh berries (strawberries, blueberries, raspberries) (1 cup)
- Granola (1/2 cup)
- Optional: Sliced almonds or chopped nuts for topping

Instructions:

1. Blend honey and Greek yogurt in a bowl until well blended.
2. Clean and prep the assortment of fresh berries.
3. Arrange the honeyed Greek yogurt, mixed fresh berries, and granola in serving glasses or bowls in an alternate pattern.
4. Continue layering until all of the glasses are full, and then top with a layer of berries.

5. For an extra crunch, you might choose to scatter chopped or sliced almonds over the top layer.

6. Present the yogurt and honey parfait right away as a tasty and nutritious dessert.

Nutritional Information (per serving):

Nutritional values may vary based on specific ingredients and quantities used.

Difficulty: Easy

A quick and healthy dessert or snack idea is this Honey and Yogurt Parfait with Fresh Berries. It's a well-balanced and enjoyable treat for youngsters, with layers of creamy Greek yogurt, sweet honey, fresh berries, and crunchy granola. This is a great dish to get youngsters involved in the preparation process because of how simple it is to put together.

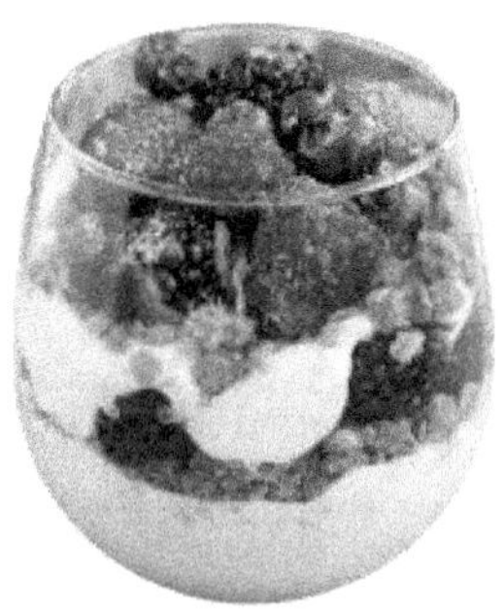

Orange and Almond Cake

Ingredients:

- Almond flour (2 cups)
- Oranges (2)
- Eggs (4)
- Honey or maple syrup (1/2 cup)
- Baking powder (1 teaspoon)
- Vanilla extract (1 teaspoon)
- Olive oil (1/4 cup)
- Optional: Sliced almonds for topping

Instructions:

1. Set the oven's temperature to 175°C/350°F. Line a circular cake pan with parchment paper and grease it.

2. After giving the oranges a good cleaning, put them whole in a saucepan of water. Once the oranges are extremely tender, bring to a boil and simmer for one to one and a half hours. Take them out of the water, let them cool, then chop them into quarters and extract the seeds.

3. Process the whole cooked orange, including the skin, in a food processor until smooth.

4. Beat the eggs and honey or maple syrup together well in a mixing basin.

5. To the egg mixture, add the blended oranges, almond flour, baking powder, vanilla essence, and olive oil. Stir until all of the ingredients are combined.

6. Transfer the mixture to the ready-made cake pan. Refine the surface with a spatula.

7. Optional: For extra texture, top the cake batter with sliced almonds.

8. Bake for about 40 to 45 minutes, or until a toothpick inserted in the middle comes out clean, in a preheated oven.

9. After letting the cake set in the pan for ten to fifteen minutes, turn it out onto a wire rack to finish cooling.

10. Slice and serve this delicious Orange and Almond Cake when it has cooled.

Nutritional Information (per serving):

Nutritional values may vary based on specific ingredients and servings.

Difficulty: Intermediate

This Orange and Almond Cake is a delicious combination of nutty almond taste and zesty citrus aromas. With its moist and rich texture, this gluten-free dessert choice is a unique and delectable treat that even young children may enjoy. There are a few phases in the preparation, but they are doable with adult supervision.

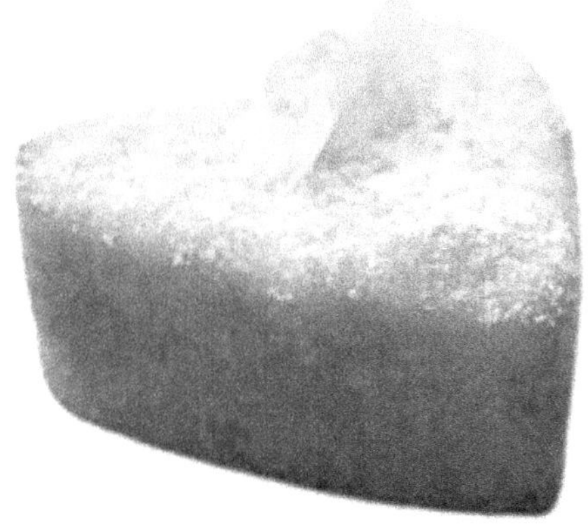

Mediterranean Fruit Salad with Citrus Mint Dressing

Ingredients:

For the Fruit Salad:

- Strawberries (sliced) (1 cup)

- Blueberries (1 cup)

- Blackberries (1 cup)

- Oranges (peeled, segmented) (2)

- Kiwi (peeled, sliced) (2)

- Grapes (halved) (1 cup)

- Pineapple (diced) (1 cup)

- Pomegranate arils (1/2 cup)

- Optional: Mint leaves for garnish

For the Citrus Mint Dressing:

- Fresh orange juice (1/4 cup)

- Fresh lemon juice (2 tablespoons)

- Honey or maple syrup (2 tablespoons)

- Fresh mint leaves (chopped) (2 tablespoons)

- Ground cinnamon (1/4 teaspoon)

- Optional: Zest of orange or lemon for extra flavor

Instructions:

1. All the prepared fruits (strawberries, blueberries, blackberries, segments oranges, sliced kiwi, split grapes, diced pineapple, and pomegranate arils) should be combined in a large mixing basin.

2. To make the citrus mint dressing, combine the fresh orange and lemon juices, honey or maple syrup, chopped fresh mint leaves, and powdered cinnamon in a separate dish. For an added burst of citrus flavor, feel free to zest an orange or lemon.

3. Toss the mixed fruits carefully to ensure they are equally coated after adding the citrus-mint dressing.

4. If you'd like, add more fresh mint leaves to the fruit salad as a garnish.

5. To allow the flavors to mingle, either serve the Mediterranean Fruit Salad right once or let it sit in the refrigerator for around half an hour.

6. Per-serving Nutritional Information:

7. The amounts and exact substances used might affect the nutritional values.

Difficulty: Easy

This zesty and delicious Mediterranean Fruit Salad with Citrus Mint Dressing makes a great snack or dessert. It is a pleasant and nutritious treat for youngsters, full of vibrant fruits complemented with a zesty citrus-mint dressing. Simple preparation lets children assist with fruit washing, chopping, and mixing under an adult's supervision.

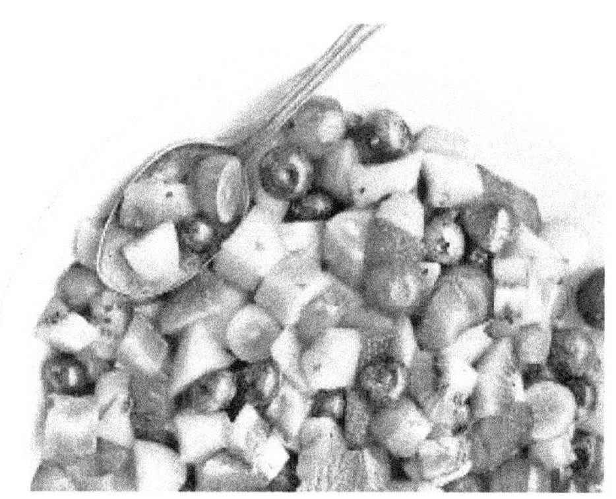

Date and Walnut Energy Balls

Ingredients:

- Dates (pitted) (1 cup)
- Walnuts (1 cup)
- Unsweetened shredded coconut (1/4 cup)
- Rolled oats (1/4 cup)
- Chia seeds (2 tablespoons)
- Honey or maple syrup (2 tablespoons)
- Vanilla extract (1 teaspoon)
- Pinch of salt

Instructions:

1. Place the walnuts and pitted dates in a food processor. Pulse till chopped finely and mixed in.

2. Process the mixture in the food processor with unsweetened shredded coconut, rolled oats, chia seeds, honey or maple syrup, vanilla essence, and a dash of salt.

3. Pulse the ingredients until everything is fully incorporated and the mixture resembles sticky dough. You may add extra honey or maple syrup or a teaspoon of water if the mixture appears too dry.

4. Using your hands, form little parts of the mixture into balls. You may choose a different size based on your preferences.

5. Transfer the date and walnut energy balls onto a parchment paper-lined plate or baking sheet.

6. The energy balls should be chilled for at least half an hour to solidify.

7. The energy balls should be refrigerated in an airtight container after they have cooled and become firm.

Nutritional Information (per serving - 2 energy balls):

Nutritional values may vary based on specific ingredients and quantities used.

Difficulty: Easy

These energy balls with dates and walnuts are a healthy and practical snack that provides you with a quick energy boost thanks to their natural ingredients, which also include oats and dates. With adult supervision, kids may help roll the ingredients into balls, making it a fun and healthful kitchen activity.

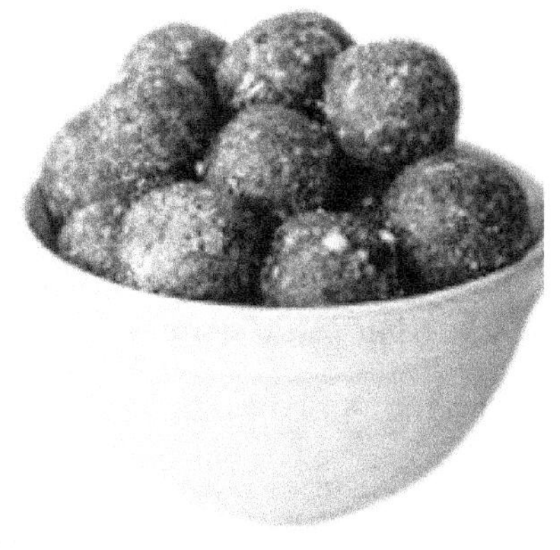

CONCLUSION

Young cooks, congrats on finishing your culinary journey with the Mediterranean Diet Cookbook for Kids! We hope that this delectable voyage has tickled your taste buds, improved your culinary abilities, and reignited your love of healthful, delicious cuisine as we conclude.

You have explored the beautiful world of Mediterranean cooking with this handbook, learning about the power of colorful veggies, lean meats, sturdy grains, and aromatic herbs. Enjoying the benefits of attentive and balanced eating, you've prepared delicious breakfasts, made filling lunches, enjoyed savory dinners, and indulged in decadent desserts.

We hope that this cookbook has given you a greater understanding of the value of a varied and nutrient-rich diet in addition to introducing you to new and fascinating tastes. By adhering to the Mediterranean Diet, you've been providing your body and mind with satisfying and healthy meals you've been doing more than simply eating.

Recall that cooking is about using your imagination, experimenting, and having fun in the kitchen—

not simply about following instructions! Every meal you've made here serves as a blank canvas for your creative culinary expression. Please feel free to add your variation, such as a dash of your preferred flavor, some herbs, or a personal touch to make it yours.

Furthermore, as you now know, the Mediterranean Diet emphasizes the communal mealtime experience in addition to the food that is placed on your plate. Food tastes better when shared with loved ones, so keep getting together with your family and friends, enjoying meals together, and cherishing these times.

Hold these culinary teachings near and dear as you progress. Take pleasure in the process of preparing meals that feed your body and spirit, enjoy the variety of tastes, and embrace the joy of cooking. Whether you're putting together lunch, putting together supper, or stirring up breakfast, never forget how much joy there is in tasting every mouthful and how much love goes into each meal you make.

Most essential, don't stop exploring! You have a vast array of tastes, cuisines, and ingredients to explore. As you experiment with new dishes, sample various fruits and vegetables, and broaden your culinary horizons, follow your curiosity. There's always something new and thrilling to learn in the kitchen, and cooking is an adventure.

So go out and explore, and may your culinary journeys be every bit as tasty and enjoyable as the dishes included in this Kids' Mediterranean Diet Cookbook.

Acknowledgment

We would like to express our sincere appreciation to all of the young chefs, parents, guardians, and mentors who accompanied us on this tasty culinary voyage as we come to a close with this Mediterranean Diet Cookbook for Kids.

Thank you very much to all of our young readers! It has been a pleasure to produce this cookbook because of your excitement, curiosity, and openness to trying new cuisines. We hope that these recipes will ignite your love of cooking, promote a balanced diet, and cultivate a taste for nutritious, delectable cuisine.

We would like to express our sincere gratitude to our readers for joining us as we explore the world of Mediterranean food. We hope that this cookbook has inspired culinary innovation, promoted mindful eating, and produced special dinner table memories.

As we get to the conclusion of our culinary voyage, keep in mind that cooking is a never-ending experience and the kitchen is your playground. Continue your exploration, experimentation, and enjoyment of delicious food and companionship.

We appreciate you coming along on this delicious journey with us. Cheers to good food and cooking!

With best wishes.

<u>Carrie Richard</u>